Keto Lunch and Side Dishes

A Vibrant Collection of Daily Keto Recipes for a Healthy Diet

By Carla Wilson

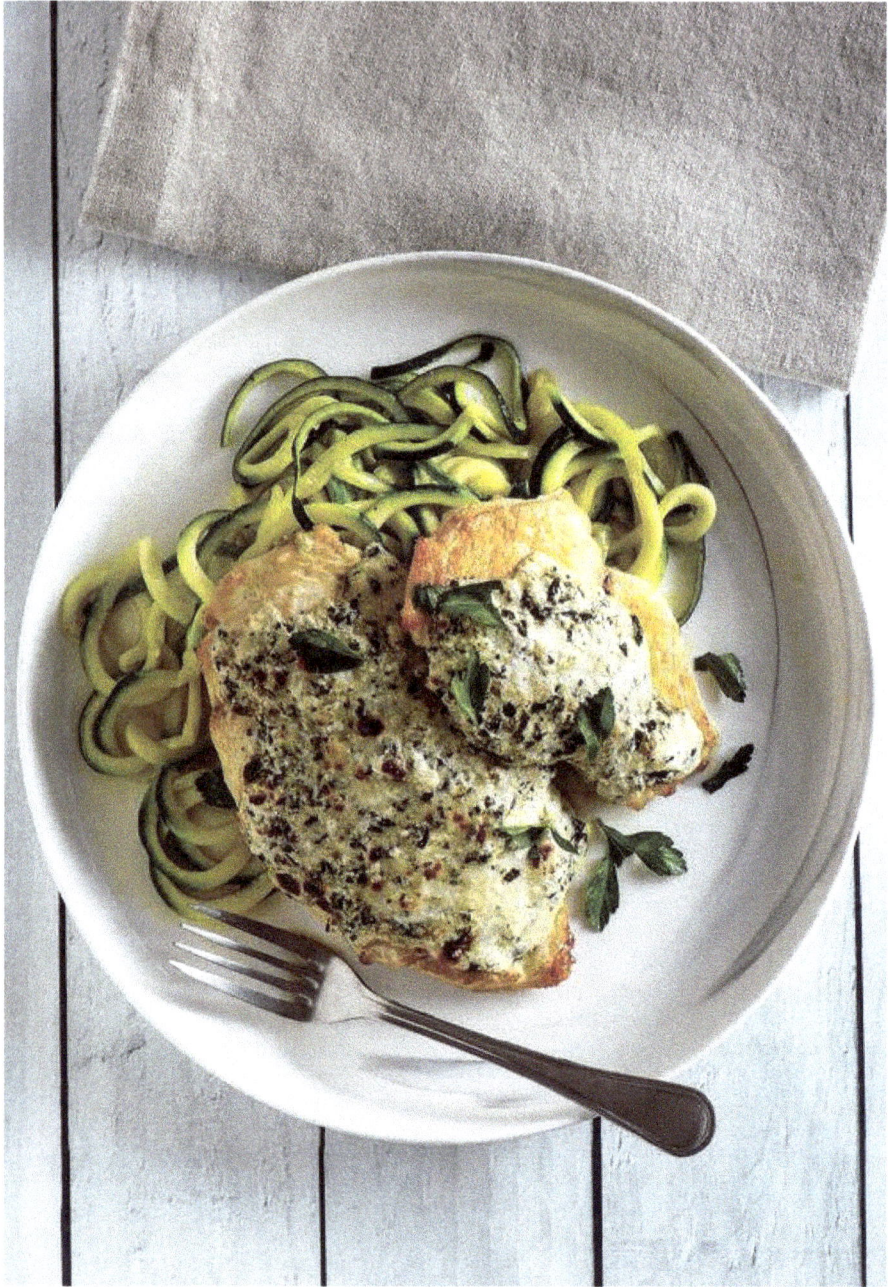

content within this book has been derived from various sources. Please consult a licensed professional before attempting any techniques outlined in this book.

By reading this document, the reader agrees that under no circumstances is the author responsible for any losses, direct or indirect, which are incurred as a result of the use of information contained within this document, including, but not limited to, — errors, omissions, or inaccuracies.

Table of Contents

Broccoli Cheese Soup.. 10

Butternut Squash Soup.. 12

Cauliflower, Leek & Bacon Soup 14

Egg Drop Soup 16

Roasted Red Pepper Soup 17

Green Chicken Enchilada Soup................................... 19

Roasted Garlic Soup... 21

French Onion Soup 23

Creamy Broccoli and Leek Soup................................. 25

Chicken Broth 27

Cream of Red Bell Pepper Soup 29

Stuffed Pepper Soup 31

Shiitake Mushroom and Asparagus Soup..................... 33

Green Chili Chicken Soup... 35

Chicken and Egg Soup 37

Vegetable Cream Soup..39

Beef and Mushroom Soup 41

Columbian Creamy Avocado Soup............................... 43

Chicken Avocado Soup 45

Hot Avocado Curry with Shrimp 47

Bacon Burger Stir Fry 49

Bacon Cheeseburger 50

Cauliflower Mac & Cheese 51

Mushroom & Cauliflower Risotto 53

Pita Pizza 54

Skillet Cabbage Tacos 55

Taco Casserole.. 57

Creamy Chicken Salad 59

Spicy Keto Chicken Wings 61

Cilantro and Lime Creamed Chicken 64

Cheesy Ham Quiche.. 66

Loaded Cauliflower Rice... 68

Creamy Garlic Chicken 69

Chinese Pork Bowl 71

Relatively Flavored Gratin.. 73

Low Carb Crack Slaw Egg Roll 75

Low Carb Beef Stir Fry.. 77

Pesto Chicken and Veggies 80

Crispy Peanut Tofu and Cauliflower Rice Stir-Fry 82

Keto Fried Chicken 84

Roasted Cauliflower with Prosciutto, Capers, and Almonds 87

Buttery Slow-Cooker Mushrooms..................................89

Baked Zucchini Gratin..91

Roasted Radishes with Brown Butter Sauce................94

Parmesan and Pork Rind Green Beans........................96

Pesto Cauliflower Steaks..98

Tomato, Avocado, and Cucumber Salad.....................100

Crunchy Pork Rind Zucchini Sticks 102

Cheese Chips and Guacamole.......................................104

Cauliflower "Potato" Salad 106

Loaded Cauliflower Mashed "Potatoes".....................109

Low Carb Broccoli and Cheese Fritters...................... 111

Broccoli Cheese Soup

Preparation Time: 20 minutes

Cooking Time: 20 minutes

Servings: 8

Ingredients

- 4 garlic cloves, minced
- 1 cup heavy cream
- 3-1/2 cups bone or chicken or vegetable broth
- 4 cups broccoli, cut into florets
- 3 cups cheddar cheese, shredded

Directions:

1. Over medium heat settings in a large pot; sauté the garlic until fragrant, for a minute.
2. Add in the chicken broth, chopped broccoli and heavy cream. Increase the heat settings and bring everything together to a boil. Once boiling; decrease the heat settings & let simmer until the broccoli is tender, for 10 to 20 minutes.
3. Slowly add in the shredded cheddar cheese & continue to cook until melted, stirring constantly, over very low heat settings (if required, work in batches and don't cook over high heat settings). Once the cheese melts

completely; immediately remove the pot from heat. Serve warm and enjoy.

Nutrition:

- 501 Calories
- 40g Total Fat
- 29g Protein

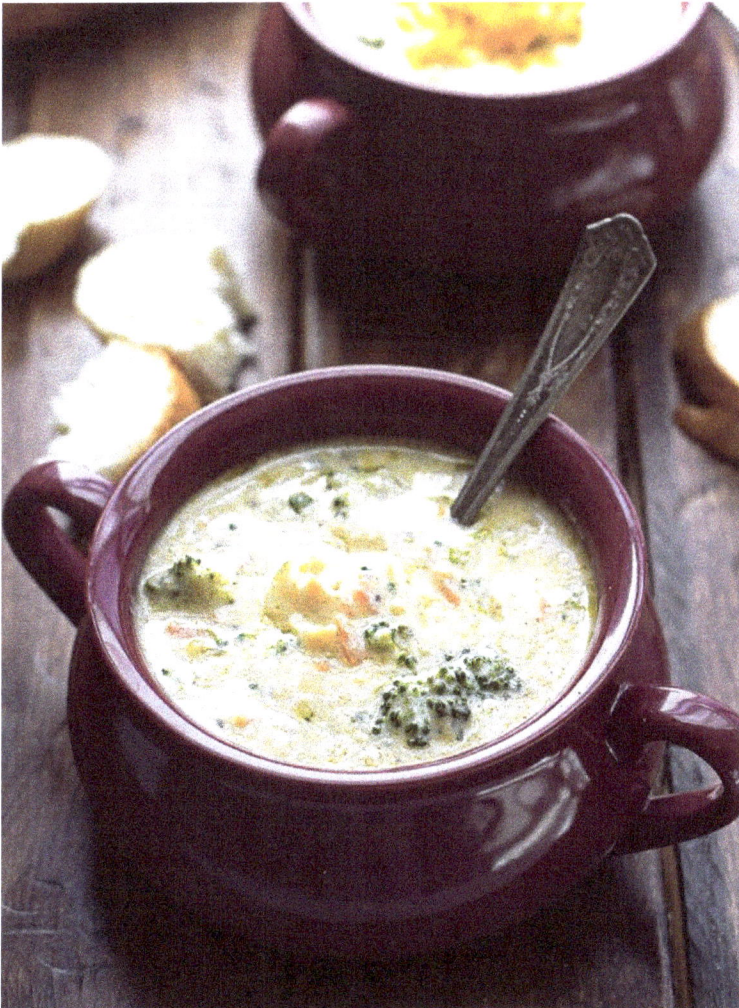

Butternut Squash Soup

Preparation Time: 15 minutes

Cooking Time: 1 hour & 10 minutes

Servings: 4

Ingredients:

- 1 tbsp. coconut oil
- 32 oz. bone or chicken broth (approximately 4 cups)
- 1 butternut squash, chopped, cut it into 1" thick slices, skin removed and cut roughly into 1" cubes
- Pepper, nutmeg & salt to taste
- 1 onion, medium-sized, roughly chopped

Directions:

1. Over low heat settings in a large pot; heat 1 tablespoon of coconut oil. Once hot; add & sauté the chopped onions until turn transparent, for a couple of minutes, stirring frequently.
2. Now, pour in the bone or chicken broth and then add in the chopped butternut squash; stir well & let simmer for an hour, over medium heat settings.
3. Now, remove the pot from heat and blend until you get a soup like consistency using an immersion blender.
4. Once pureed, season the soup with pepper, nutmeg & salt to taste.

5. Stir well and cook for 30 more minutes. Serve warm and enjoy

Nutrition:

- 72 Calories
- 4g Total Fat
- 2.2g Protein

Cauliflower, Leek & Bacon Soup

Preparation Time: 10 minutes

Cooking Time: 2 hours & 10 minutes

Servings: 4

Ingredients:

- 4 cups vegetable or chicken broth
- 1/2 head of cauliflower; cut into small pieces
- 5 bacon strips
- 1 leek; cut into small pieces
- Pepper and salt to taste

Directions:

1. Place the leek and cauliflower pieces into a large pot and then fill the pot with chicken broth. Bring it to a boil over moderate heat settings until tender, for 1 to 1-1/2 hours. To create a smooth soup; puree the vegetables using an immersion blender.

2. Microwave the bacon strips on high-heat settings for a minute and then cut into small pieces; dropping the pieces into the soup. Cook for 30 more minutes on low-heat settings. Add pepper and salt to taste

Nutrition:

- 222 Calories
- 15g Total Fat
- 8.5g Protein

Egg Drop Soup

Preparation Time: 10 minutes

Cooking Time: 20 minutes

Servings: 2

Ingredients:

- A pinch of red pepper flakes
- 4 cups bone broth or 2 large bouillon cubes plus 4 cups of water
- Freshly ground pepper
- 2 eggs, large

Directions:

1. Scramble the eggs with some fresh pepper in a large bowl; set aside.
2. Now, over high heat settings in a small pot; add bone broth & a pinch of red pepper flakes. Bring it to a boil and then, slowly stir in the egg mixture; continue to mix and bring it to a boil again.

Nutrition:

- 75 Calories
- 4.8g Total Fat
- 6.4g Protein

Roasted Red Pepper Soup

Preparation Time: 15 minutes

Cooking Time: 40 minutes

Servings: 8

Ingredients:

- 1-pound cauliflower rice or cauliflower, chopped
- 2-1/2 pounds sweet peppers
- 1-1/2 tsp. sweetener
- 2 cups half and half
- 1-1/2 tsp. salt
- 2 cups chicken or vegetable broth

Directions:

1. Arrange the sweet peppers in a single layer on a large-sized baking sheet & roast until softened & browned slightly, for half an hour, at 400 F.
2. In the meantime, add the broth & cauliflower to a large stock pot. Let simmer until the peppers are done, over medium heat settings.
3. Add in the cauliflower, peppers, half the broth & the leftover ingredients to a blender. Blend until smooth, for a minute or two. Add the mixture to the pot again & cook until heated through

Nutrition:

- 254 Calories
- 16g Total Fat
- 14g Protein

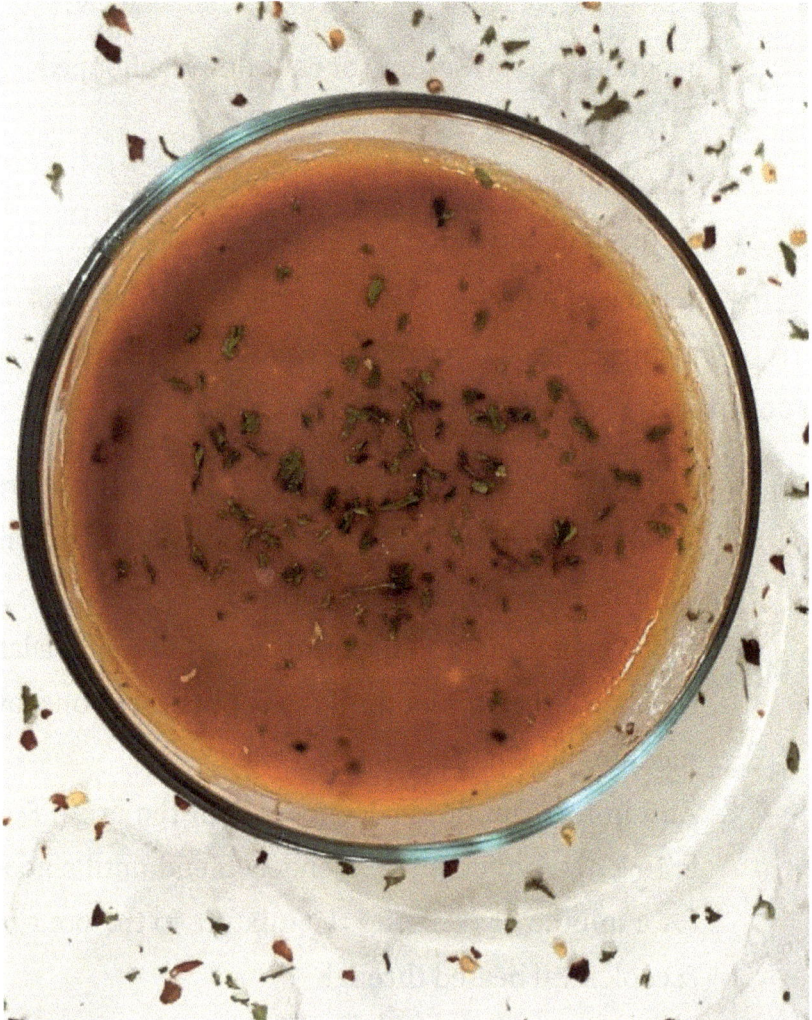

Green Chicken Enchilada Soup

Preparation Time: 10 minutes

Cooking Time: 20 minutes

Servings: 4

Ingredients:

- 1 tsp. garlic powder
- 1/2-pound Brussels sprouts, thinly sliced
- Caesar dressing, for dipping
- 2 tbsp. freshly grated parmesan
- 1 tbsp. olive oil

Directions:

1. Combine cream cheese together with salsa, chicken stock and cheddar cheese in a blender; blend on high settings until completely smooth.
2. Pour the mixture into a saucepan, preferably medium-sized & cook on medium heat settings until hot; ensure you don't bring it to a boil.
3. Add in the shredded chicken; cook until heated through, for 3 to 5 more minutes.
4. Garnish with more of shredded cheddar & chopped cilantro. Serve immediately and enjoy.

Nutrition:

- 108 Calories
- 8.6g Total Fat
- 2.9g Protein

Roasted Garlic Soup

Preparation Time: 15 minutes

Cooking Time: 20 minutes

Servings: 6

Ingredients:

- 1 head of cauliflower, large, chopped (roughly 5 cups)
- 2 bulbs of garlic; outer layers peeled but keeping the individual cloves intact; further cutting it into 1/4" from the top
- 6 cups gluten-free vegetable broth
- 1 tbsp. extra-virgin olive oil, divided
- 3 shallots, chopped
- Freshly ground pepper & sea salt, to taste

Directions:

1. Preheat your oven to 400 F in advance. Place the garlic bulb on a square of aluminum foil & coat with 1/2 tsp. of olive oil. Heat in the prepared oven roughly for half an hour.
2. Once done, let it cool slightly. Remove the aluminum foil & squeezing the garlic out from each clove.
3. In the meantime, pour the leftover olive oil in a saucepan, preferably medium-sized. Heat over medium-high heat settings & add in the chopped

shallots; sauté for 4 to 6 minutes, until tender & starting to turn brown.

4. Add in roasted garlic together with leftover ingredients to the saucepan. Cover & bring everything together to a boil. Once boiling; decrease the heat settings to low & let simmer until the cauliflower is softened, for 15 to 20 more minutes.

5. Drop the mixture into the blender or food processor. Puree on high settings until smooth. Sprinkle pepper and salt to taste. Serve & enjoy.

Nutrition:

- 73 Calories
- 2.7g Total Fat
- 2.9g Protein

French Onion Soup

Preparation Time: 20 minutes

Cooking Time: 45 minutes

Servings: 6

Ingredients:

- 4 drops erythritol or stevia/2 tsp. Native or Erythritol
- 1-1/4 pounds medium-sized brown onion; chopped
- 5 tbsp. Butter
- 3 cup Beef stock
- 4 tbsp. olive oil

Directions:

1. Over medium low heat settings in a pot, preferably medium to large sized heat the olive oil and butter. Once melted; add in the onions & 1 tsp. of salt.
2. Cook until the onions turn golden brown, for 20 minutes, uncovered, stirring frequently. Stir in the stevia & cook for 5 more minutes.
3. Add stock to the saucepan; decrease the heat settings to low & let simmer for 25 more minutes.
4. Ladle the soup into separate soup bowls; serve immediately and enjoy.

Nutrition:

- 218 Calories
- 19g Total Fat
- 3.5g Protein

Creamy Broccoli and Leek Soup

Preparation Time: 10 minutes

Cooking Time: 20 minutes

Servings: 4

Ingredients:

- 10 oz. broccoli; cut the core off & thinly sliced; divide the remaining into small florets
- 1 leek; thoroughly rinsed & finely chopped
- 8 oz. cream cheese
- 1/2 cup basil, fresh
- 3 cups water
- 1 clove garlic
- 3 oz. olive oil
- Pepper and salt to taste

Directions:

1. Place the sliced broccoli core and leek in a pot; fill with water (enough to cover). Season with salt & bring everything together to a boil on high heat settings until the broccoli stem can be easily pierced using a knife, for a couple of minutes.
2. Add in the florets & garlic. Decrease the heat settings & let simmer until the broccoli is tender and turns bright green, for a couple of more minutes.

3. Add in the cream cheese, olive oil, basil and freshly ground black pepper. Blend the soup using an immersion blender until you get your desired consistency. Serve and enjoy.

Nutrition:

- 482 Calories
- 30g Total Fat
- 46g Protein

Chicken Broth

Preparation Time: 15 minutes

Cooking Time: 8 hours & 10 minutes

Servings: 10

Ingredients:

- 20 fresh basil leaves (10 for the slow cooker, and 10 for garnish)
- One whole chicken
- 5 thick slices of ginger, fresh
- A stalk of fresh lemongrass, cut into large chunks
- 1 medium lime
- Salt to taste

Directions:

1. Place chicken together with ginger, 10 basil leaves, lemongrass & salt into the bottom of your slow cooker. Add water to your slow cooker.
2. Cook for 8 to 10 hours on low-heat settings. Ladle the broth into a large bowl or pitcher; add salt to taste & squeeze in the fresh lime juice. Garnish the broth with fresh chopped basil leaves.

Nutrition:

- 357 Calories
- 15g Total Fat
- 43g Protein

Cream of Red Bell Pepper Soup

Preparation Time: 10 minutes

Cooking Time: 30 minutes

Servings: 4

Ingredients:

- 2 ½ pounds red bell peppers
- 4 tablespoons of coconut oil
- 2 shallots
- medium garlic cloves
- cups of homemade low-sodium vegetable stock
- 2 teaspoons red wine vinegar
- ½ teaspoon cayenne pepper
- 1 teaspoon salt
- 1 teaspoon black pepper
- ½ cup of heavy cream

Directions:

1. Click "Sauté" function in Pressure Pot and add the coconut oil. Once hot, add the bell peppers, shallots, and garlic cloves. Sauté until softened.
2. Stir in remaining ingredients except for the heavy cream.
3. Seal and set at high pressure for 3 minutes. When done, quickly release the tension and carefully remove

the cover. Blend the soup. Stir in heavy cream and season.

Nutrition:

- 302 calories
- 12g fat
- 39g protein

Stuffed Pepper Soup

Preparation Time: 10 minutes

Cooking Time: 35 minutes

Servings: 6

Ingredients:

- 1 lb. lean ground beef
- 2 tbsp. coconut oil
- small onion
- large red bell peppers
- 1 (28-ounce) can tomatoes
- (14.5-ounce) can tomato sauce
- cups of homemade low-sodium chicken stock
- 2 cups of cauliflower rice
- 1 teaspoon garlic powder

Directions.

1. Press the "Sauté" function on your Pressure Pot and add the coconut oil, ground beef, bell peppers, and onions.
2. Add the remaining ingredients and stir. Cover and set at high pressure for 15 minutes. When done, release the pressure and slowly take off the lid.
3. Stir the soup again. Serve!

Nutrition:

- 304 calories
- 10g fat
- 38g protein

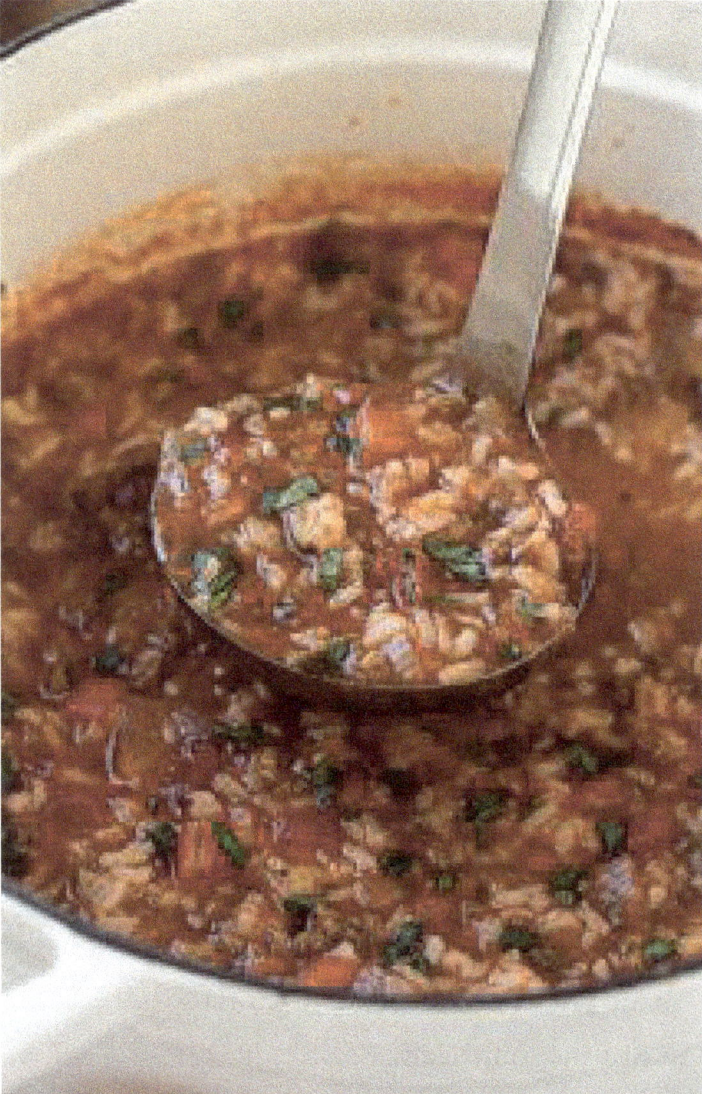

Shiitake Mushroom and Asparagus Soup

Preparation Time: 10 minutes

Cooking Time: 35 minutes

Servings: 4

Ingredients:

- 1 pound of asparagus
- 1 pound of shiitake mushrooms
- 4 cups of baby spinach
- 4 tablespoons of coconut oil
- 4 cups low-sodium chicken stock
- 1 bay leaf
- 1 cup of heavy cream
- ¼ cup of fresh parsley
- 1 lemon
- 1 teaspoon salt
- 1 teaspoon black pepper

Directions:

1. Set your Pressure Pot on "Sauté" and stir in coconut oil. Once hot, add the onions and garlic cloves. Sauté until translucent.
2. Sauté chopped mushrooms and asparagus for 3 minutes.

3. Incorporate rest of ingredients except for the heavy cream. Close and cook at high pressure for 15 minutes. When done, allow for a full original release pressure method and carefully remove the cover. Mix in the heavy cream. Serve!

Nutrition:

- 315 calories
- 12g fat
- 36g protein

Green Chili Chicken Soup

Preparation Time: 10 minutes

Cooking Time: 40 minutes

Servings: 6

Ingredients:

- 3 chicken breasts
- red bell pepper
- tablespoons of coconut oil
- 1 onion
- celery stalks
- garlic cloves
- 4 cups of homemade low-sodium chicken stock
- (16-ounce) jar of salsa Verde
- (4-ounce) cans of diced green chilies
- 1 tablespoon ground cumin
- 1 tablespoon oregano
- 1 teaspoon salt
- 1 teaspoon black pepper
- ¼ cup of fresh cilantro

Directions:

1. Select "Sauté" function on Pressure Pot and pour coconut oil. Once hot, mix in chicken breasts and sear on both sides.
2. Gently stir in the remaining ingredients. Close and cook in high pressure for 15 minutes. When done, allow for a full natural release method. Carefully remove the cover.
3. Transfer chicken in a cutting board and shred using two forks. Stir the shredded chicken into the soup.

Nutrition:

- 314 calories
- 16g fat
- 39g protein

Chicken and Egg Soup

Preparation Time: 10 minutes

Cooking Time: 15 minutes

Servings: 4

Ingredients:

- 2 cups of homemade low-sodium chicken stock
- large organic eggs
- 3 fresh scallions
- 1 teaspoon sesame oil
- 1 tablespoon ginger
- 1 teaspoon garlic powder
- 1 teaspoon salt
- 1 teaspoon black pepper
- 1 teaspoon xanthan gum
- A drop of yellow food coloring.

Directions:

1. Add all the ingredients inside your Pressure Pot except for the arrowroot powder and give a good stir.
2. Close and cook in high pressure for 3 minutes. When done, naturally release the tension and carefully remove the cover. Stir in the yellow food coloring and arrowroot powder.
3. Cook until the liquid thickens. Serve and enjoy!

Nutrition:

- 320 calories
- 15g fat
- 37g protein

Vegetable Cream Soup

Preparation Time: 10 minutes

Cooking Time: 35 minutes

Servings: 6

Ingredients:

- 1-pound cauliflower florets
- 1-pound broccoli florets
- bunch of kale
- celery ribs
- 4 tablespoons of extra-virgin olive oil
- 2 medium garlic cloves
- 1 medium red onion,
- 10 cups of homemade low-sodium vegetable stock
- 1 cup of heavy cream
- 1 teaspoon salt
- 1 tablespoon of Dijon mustard
- 1 tablespoon of fresh parsley

Directions:

1. Press the "Sauté" function on your Pressure Pot and add the olive oil. Once hot, add the onions and garlic cloves. Sauté until translucent, stirring frequently.
2. Add the celery, cauliflower florets, and broccoli florets. Cook for 2 minutes

3. Add the remaining ingredients except for the heavy cream inside your Pressure Pot. Close the lid and select at high pressure for 15 minutes. When done, naturally release the tension and carefully remove the cover.

4. Puree the soup until smooth. Gently stir in the heavy cream. Serve and enjoy!

Nutrition:

- 324 calories
- 16g fat
- 34g protein

Beef and Mushroom Soup

Preparation Time: 10 minutes

Cooking Time: 25 minutes

Servings: 4

Ingredients:

- 1 pound of ground beef
- a pound of mushrooms
- tablespoons of coconut oil
- 1 small onion
- 4 garlic cloves
- 1 teaspoon salt
- 1 teaspoon black paper
- 2 cups homemade low-sodium beef broth

Directions:

1. Press "Sauté" in Pressure Pot and fill coconut oil. Once hot, add the ground beef, onions, and garlic. Cook until the brown, stirring occasionally. Mix in remaining ingredients and lock the lid.
2. Cook at high pressure for 12 minutes. When done, release the tension and carefully remove the cover. Stir the soup again and adjust the seasoning if necessary. Serve and enjoy!

Nutrition:

- 327 calories
- 17g fat
- 38g protein

Columbian Creamy Avocado Soup

Preparation Time: 10 minutes

Cooking Time: 20 minutes

Servings: 4

Ingredients:

- 4 tablespoons avocado oil
- 1 shallot
- 1 garlic clove
- 4 cups of homemade low-sodium chicken stock
- 4 medium ripe avocados
- tablespoon lime juice
- cups heavy cream
- 1 teaspoon salt
- 1 teaspoon black pepper
- ¼ cup of fresh cilantro

Directions:

1. Press the "Sauté" and add the avocado oil. Once hot, add the chopped shallots and minced garlic. Sauté for 3 minutes, stirring frequently.
2. Add the chicken stock, lime juice, avocados, and seasonings. Close the lid and set in high pressure for 3 minutes. When done, release tension and remove the cover.

43

3. Puree the soup until smooth. Stir in the heavy cream and fresh cilantro.

Nutrition:

- 317 calories
- 16g fat
- 39g protein

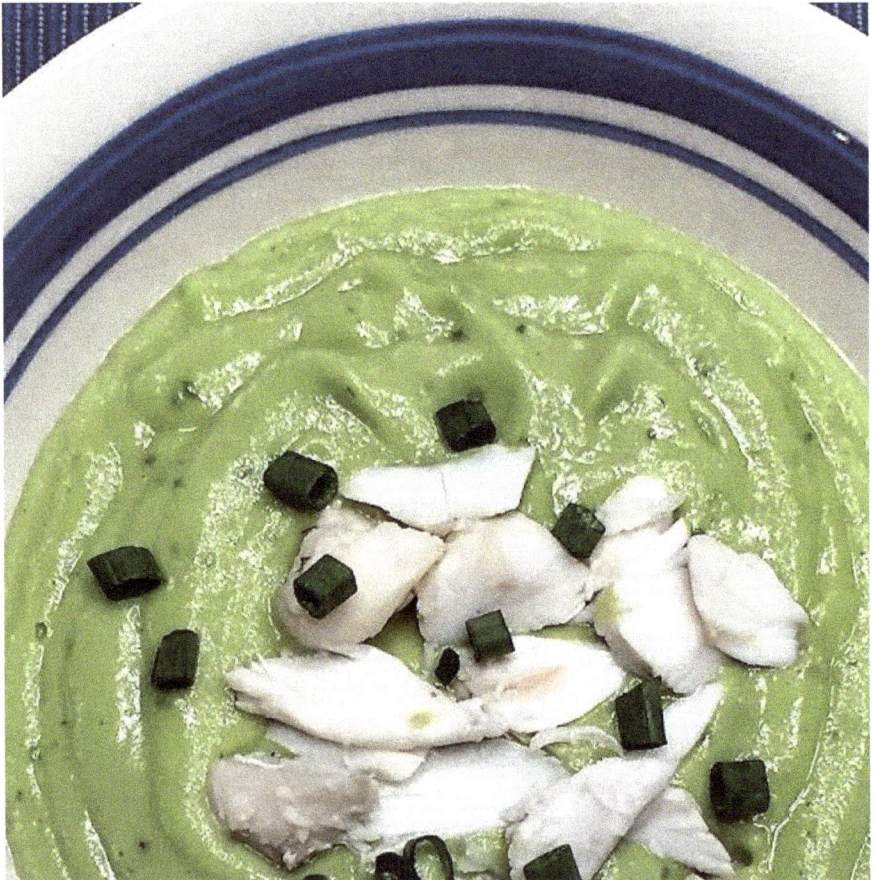

Chicken Avocado Soup

Preparation Time: 10 minutes

Cooking Time: 20 minutes

Servings: 4

Ingredients:

- 2 pounds chicken thighs
- 1 green onion
- 1 jalapeno pepper
- 4 cups homemade low-sodium chicken stock
- 2 tablespoons olive oil
- 6 garlic cloves
- 2 teaspoons cumin
- ½ cup of fresh cilantro
- 2 lime juice
- large avocados

Directions:

1. Press the "Sauté" Pressure Pot and add the olive oil. Once hot, place the chicken thighs and sear for 4 minutes.
2. Add in the remaining ingredients except for heavy cream and avocados. Close and cook at high pressure for 8 minutes. When done, quickly release the tension

and remove the cover. Place the chicken in a cutting board and shred using two forks.

3. Use immersion blender into Pressure Pot. Stir in the mashed avocados, heavy cream, and shredded chicken.

Nutrition:

- 317 calories
- 18g fat
- 37g protein

Hot Avocado Curry with Shrimp

Preparation Time: 10 minutes

Cooking Time: 20 minutes

Servings: 2

Ingredients:

- ½ pound of shrimp
- 2 cups low-sodium chicken stock
- (14-ounce) can of coconut milk
- avocados, ripe
- ½ teaspoon cayenne pepper
- 1 teaspoon salt
- 1 tablespoon lime juice

Directions:

1. Blend all the ingredients except for the shrimp. Pour in the mixture inside your Pressure Pot with the shrimp.
2. Lock and cook at high pressure for 3 minutes. When done, quickly release the tension and remove the cover.

Nutrition:

- 317 calories
- 12g fat
- 38g protein

Bacon Burger Stir Fry

Preparation Time: 10 minutes

Cooking Time: 20 minutes

Servings: 10

Ingredients:

- 1 lb. Ground beef
- 1 lb. Bacon
- 1 Small onion
- 3 garlic cloves
- 1 Cabbage

Directions:

1. Dice the bacon and onion. Mix the beef and bacon in a wok.
2. Mince the onion and garlic. Toss both into the hot grease. Slice and toss in the cabbage and stir-fry. Mix in the meat and season.

Nutrition:

- 32g Protein
- 22g Fats
- 357 Calories

Bacon Cheeseburger

Preparation Time: 15 minutes

Cooking Time: 30 minutes

Servings: 12

Ingredients:

- 16 oz. Low-sodium bacon
- 3 lb. Ground beef
- 2 Eggs
- ½ Medium onion
- 8 oz. cheddar cheese

Directions:

1. Fry the bacon and chop it to bits. Shred the cheese and dice the onion. Mix the mixture with the beef and whisked eggs.
2. Grill 24 burger if desired.

Nutrition:

- 27g Protein
- 41g Fats
- 489 Calories

Cauliflower Mac & Cheese

Preparation Time: 15 minutes

Cooking Time: 20 minutes

Servings: 4

Ingredients:

- 1 Cauliflower
- 3 tbsp. Butter
- ¼ cup unsweetened almond milk
- ¼ cup Heavy cream
- 1 cup Cheddar cheese

Directions:

1. Slice the cauliflower into small florets. Shred the cheese. Prepare the oven to 450° Fahrenheit. Wrap baking pan with foil.
2. Melt two tablespoons butter. Mix the florets, butter, salt, and pepper. Roast the cauliflower on the baking pan for 15 minutes.
3. Warm rest of the butter, milk, heavy cream, and cheese in the microwave. Pour the cheese and serve.

Nutrition:

- 11g Protein
- 23g Fats
- 294 Calories

Mushroom & Cauliflower Risotto

Preparation Time: 5 minutes

Cooking Time: 10 minutes

Servings: 4

Ingredients:

- 1 cauliflower
- 1 cup Vegetable stock
- 9 oz. mushrooms
- 2 tbsp. Butter
- 1 cup Coconut cream

Directions:

1. Pour the stock in a saucepan. Boil and set aside. Prepare a skillet with butter and sauté the mushrooms.
2. Grate and stir in the cauliflower and stock. Simmer and add the cream. Serve.

Nutrition:

- 1g Protein
- 17g Fats
- 186 Calories

Pita Pizza

Preparation Time: 15 minutes

Cooking Time: 10 minutes

Servings: 2

Ingredients:

- ½ cup Marinara sauce
- 1 Low-carb pita
- 2 oz. Cheddar cheese
- 14 Pepperoni slices
- 1 oz. Roasted red peppers

Directions:

1. Set oven to 450° Fahrenheit.
2. Slice the pita in half and place onto a foil-lined baking tray. Rub with a bit of oil and toast for 2 minutes.
3. Pour the sauce over the bread. Sprinkle using the cheese and other toppings. Bake for 5 minutes.

Nutrition:

- 13g Protein
- 19g Fats
- 250 Calories

Skillet Cabbage Tacos

Preparation Time: 10 minutes

Cooking Time: 15 minutes

Servings: 4

Ingredients:

- 1 lb. Ground beef
- ½ cup Salsa
- 2 cups cabbage
- 2 tsp. Chili powder
- ¾ cup cheese

Directions:

1. Brown the beef and drain the fat. Pour in the salsa, cabbage, and seasoning.
2. Cover and lower the heat. Simmer 12 minutes using the medium heat.
3. Once softened, remove it from the heat and mix in the cheese.
4. Top with green onions.

Nutrition:

- 30g Protein
- 21g Fats
- 325 Calories

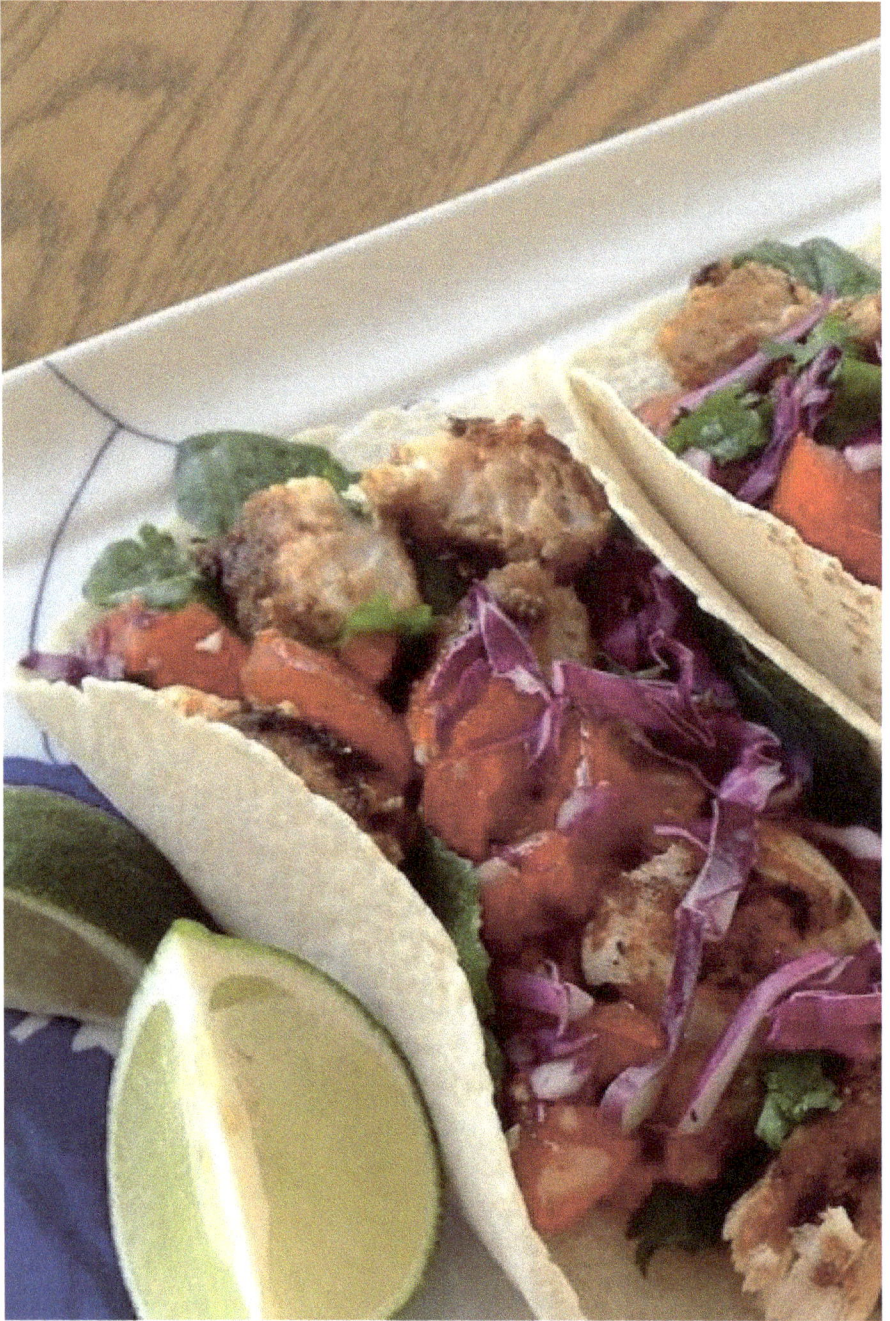

Taco Casserole

Preparation Time: 10 minutes

Cooking Time: 20 minutes

Servings: 8

Ingredients:

- 2 lbs. Ground beef
- 2 tbsp. Taco seasoning
- 8 oz. cheddar cheese
- 1 cup Salsa
- 16 oz. Cottage cheese

Directions:

1. Heat the oven to 400° Fahrenheit.
2. Combine the taco seasoning and ground meat in a casserole dish. Bake for 20 minutes.
3. Combine the salsa and both kinds of cheese. Set aside.
4. Drain away the cooking juices from the meat.
5. Mash the meat into small pieces.
6. Sprinkle with cheese. Bake in the oven for 20.

Nutrition:

- 45g Protein
- 18g Fats
- 367 Calories

Creamy Chicken Salad

Preparation Time: 10 minutes

Cooking Time: 30 minutes

Servings: 4

Ingredients:

- 1 lb. Chicken Breast
- 2 Avocados
- 2 Garlic Cloves
- 3 tbsp. Lime Juice
- 1/3 cup Onion
- 1 Jalapeno Pepper
- 1 tbsp. Cilantro

Directions

1. Set oven to 400 F. Line cooking sheet with foil. Layer the chicken breast up with some olive oil before seasoning.
2. Situate onto cooking sheet and put into the oven for 20 minutes. Let it cool and shred. Combine everything into a bowl and mash the avocado. Season well!

Nutrition:

- 20g Fats
- 4g Carbohydrates
- 25g Protein

Spicy Keto Chicken Wings

Preparation Time: 20 Minutes

Cooking Time: 30 minutes

Servings: 4

Ingredients:

- 2 lbs. Chicken Wings
- 1 tsp. Cajun Spice
- 2 tsp. Smoked Paprika
- ½ tsp. Turmeric
- 2 tsp. Baking Powder

Directions:

1. Prep the stove to 400 F. Dry chicken wings with a paper towel.
2. Mix all of the seasonings along with the baking powder. Toss the chicken wings in and coat evenly. Put on a wire rack that is placed over your baking tray.
3. Cook for 30 minutes. Pull out from the oven and flip to bake the other side for 30 minutes.
4. Take it out and set aside. Serve.

Nutrition:

- 7g Fats
- 1g Carbohydrates
- 60g Proteins

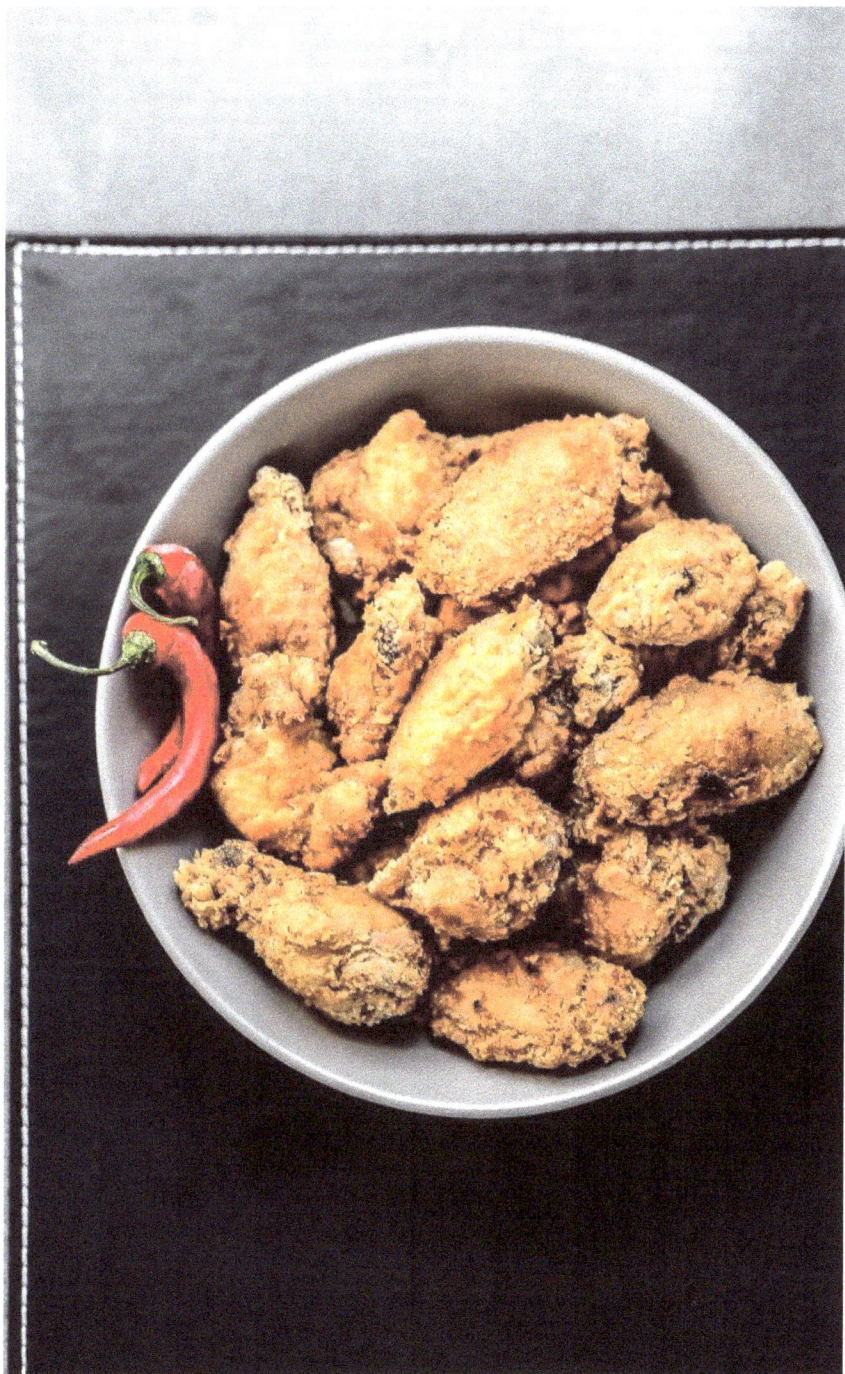

Cilantro and Lime Creamed Chicken

Preparation Time: 10 Minutes

Cooking Time: 20 minutes

Servings: 4

Ingredients:

- 4 Chicken Breast
- 1 tsp. Red Pepper Flakes
- 1 tbsp. Cilantro
- 2 tbsp. Lime Juice
- 1 cup Chicken Broth
- ¼ cup Onion
- 1 tbsp. Olive Oil
- ½ cup Heavy Cream

Directions:

1. Preheat skillet and place it over a moderate temperature. Season the chicken breast. Throw into the skillet and cook for 8 minutes on each side. Set aside

2. Stir in the onion and cook them for a minute then mix in cilantro, pepper flakes, lime juice, and the chicken broth.

3. Boil for 10 minutes. Whisk in your heavy cream and add in the chicken to coat.

Nutrition:

- 20g Fats
- 6g Carbohydrates
- 30g Proteins

Cheesy Ham Quiche

Preparation Time: 10 minutes

Cooking Time: 30 minutes

Servings: 6

Ingredients:

- 8 Eggs
- 1 cup Zucchini
- ½ cup heavy Cream
- 1 cup Ham
- 1 tsp. Mustard

Directions:

1. Prep stove to 375 and get pie plate for your quiche. Shred the zucchini.

2. Once done, drain. Place the zucchini into your pie plate along with the cooked ham pieces and cheese. Whisk the seasonings, cream, and eggs. Pour on top then cook for 40 minutes.

3. If the quiche is cooked to your liking, take the dish from the oven and allow it to chill slightly before slicing.

Nutrition:

- 25g Fats
- 2g Carbohydrates
- 20g Proteins

Loaded Cauliflower Rice

Preparation Time: 10 minutes

Cooking Time: 20 minutes

Servings: 4

Ingredients:

- 1 Cauliflower
- 1 cup Cheddar Cheese
- 1 lb. Bacon
- ½ cup Chives

Directions:

1. Rice your cauliflower. You can choose to do this by hand. Cook the bacon in a grilling pan over a medium heat.
2. Place your cauliflower rice into a microwave-safe bowl and sprinkle your shredded cheese over the top.
3. Place bowl into the microwave for a minute and allow for the rice to cook through and the cheese to melt.
4. Top with your bacon pieces and season to your liking.

Nutrition:

- 10g Fats
- 5g Carbohydrates
- 5g Proteins

Creamy Garlic Chicken

Preparation Time: 5 minutes

Cooking Time: 15 minutes

Servings: 4

Ingredients:

- 4 chicken breasts
- 1 tsp. garlic powder
- 1 tsp. paprika
- 2 tbsp. butter
- 1 tsp. salt
- 1 cup heavy cream
- ½ cup sun-dried tomatoes
- 2 cloves garlic
- 1 cup spinach

Directions:

1. Blend the paprika, garlic powder, and salt and rub both sides of the chicken.
2. Melt the butter in a frying pan over medium heat. Fry chicken for 5 minutes each side. Set aside.
3. Whisk the heavy cream, sun-dried tomatoes, and garlic. Cook for 2 minutes. Sauté spinach for additional 3 minutes. Place chicken back to the pan and cover with the sauce.

Nutrition:

- 12g Carbohydrates
- 26g Fat
- 4g Protein

Chinese Pork Bowl

Preparation Time: 5 minutes

Cooking Time: 15 minutes

Servings: 4

Ingredients:

- 1¼ pounds pork belly
- 2 Tbsp. tamari soy sauce
- 1 Tbsp. rice vinegar
- 2 cloves garlic
- 3 oz. butter
- 1-pound Brussels sprouts
- ½ leek

Directions:

1. Fry the pork over medium-high heat.
2. Combine the garlic cloves, butter, and Brussels sprouts. Add in to the pan and cook.
3. Drizzle soy sauce and rice vinegar together and pour into the pan. Season.
4. Top with chopped leek.

Nutrition:

- 7g Carbohydrates
- 97g Protein
- 993 Calories

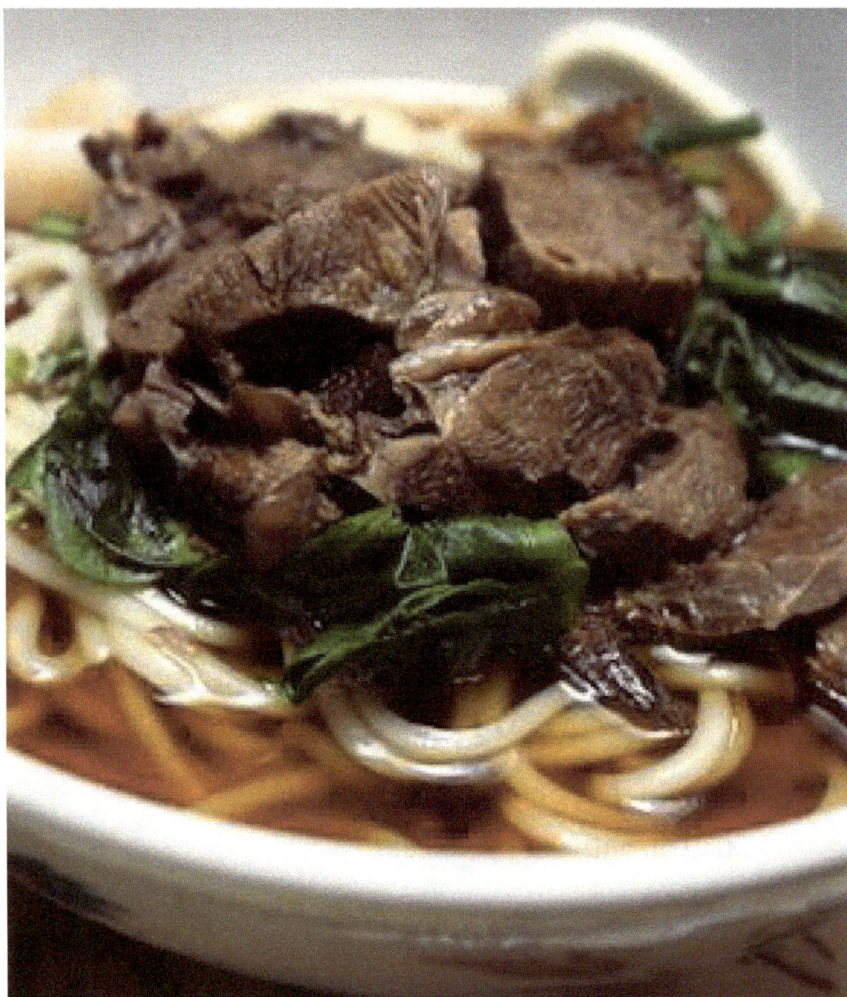

Relatively Flavored Gratin

Preparation Time: 15 minutes

Cooking Time: 46 minutes

Servings: 8

Ingredients:

- ½ C. heavy whipping cream
- 2 tbsp. butter
- ½ tsp. garlic powder
- ¼ tsp. xanthan gum
- 4 C. zucchini
- 1 small yellow onion
- 1½ C. pepper jack cheese

Directions:

1. Prepare oven to 375 0 F and grease a 9×9-inch baking dish. In a microwave-safe dish, mix heavy whipping cream, butter, garlic powder, and xanthan gum and melt 1 minute.

2. Arrange 1/3 of zucchini and onion slices at the bottom and season and ½ C. of pepper jack cheese. Repeat the layers twice. Spread the cream mixture on top evenly. Bake for 45 minutes. Remove the baking dish from oven and set aside.

Nutrition:

- 140 Calories
- 3.9g Carbohydrates
- 5.5g Protein

Low Carb Crack Slaw Egg Roll

Preparation time: 10 minutes

Cooking Time: 20 minutes

Serving: 2

Ingredients:

- 1 lb. ground beef
- 4 cups shredded coleslaw mix
- 1 tbsp. avocado oil
- 1 tsp. sea salt
- ¼ tsp. black pepper
- 4 cloves garlic, minced
- 3 tbsp. fresh ginger, grated
- ¼ cup coconut amines
- 2 tsp. toasted sesame oil
- ¼ cup green onions

Directions:

1. Cook avocado oil over medium-high heat. Cook the garlic.
2. Cook ground beef for 10 minutes. Season well.
3. Once cooked, you can lower the heat and add the coleslaw mix and the coconut amines. Stir for 5 minutes.
4. Garnish green onions and the toasted sesame oil.

Nutrition:

- 104 calories
- 5g fat
- 18g protein

Low Carb Beef Stir Fry

Preparation Time: 10 minutes

Cooking Time: 25 minutes

Serving: 3

Ingredients:

- ½ cup zucchini
- ¼ cup organic broccoli florets
- 1 bunch baby bok choy
- 2 tbsp. avocado oil
- 2 tsp. coconut amines
- 1 small ginger
- 8 oz. skirt steak

Directions:

1. Heat the pan and add 1 tbsp. oil. Sear steak on high heat for 2 minutes per side.
2. Set to medium heat and cook the broccoli, ginger, ghee, and coconut amines.
3. Cook the book choy for another minute
4. Mix in zucchini and cook.

Nutrition:

- 104 calories
- 6g fat
- 31g protein

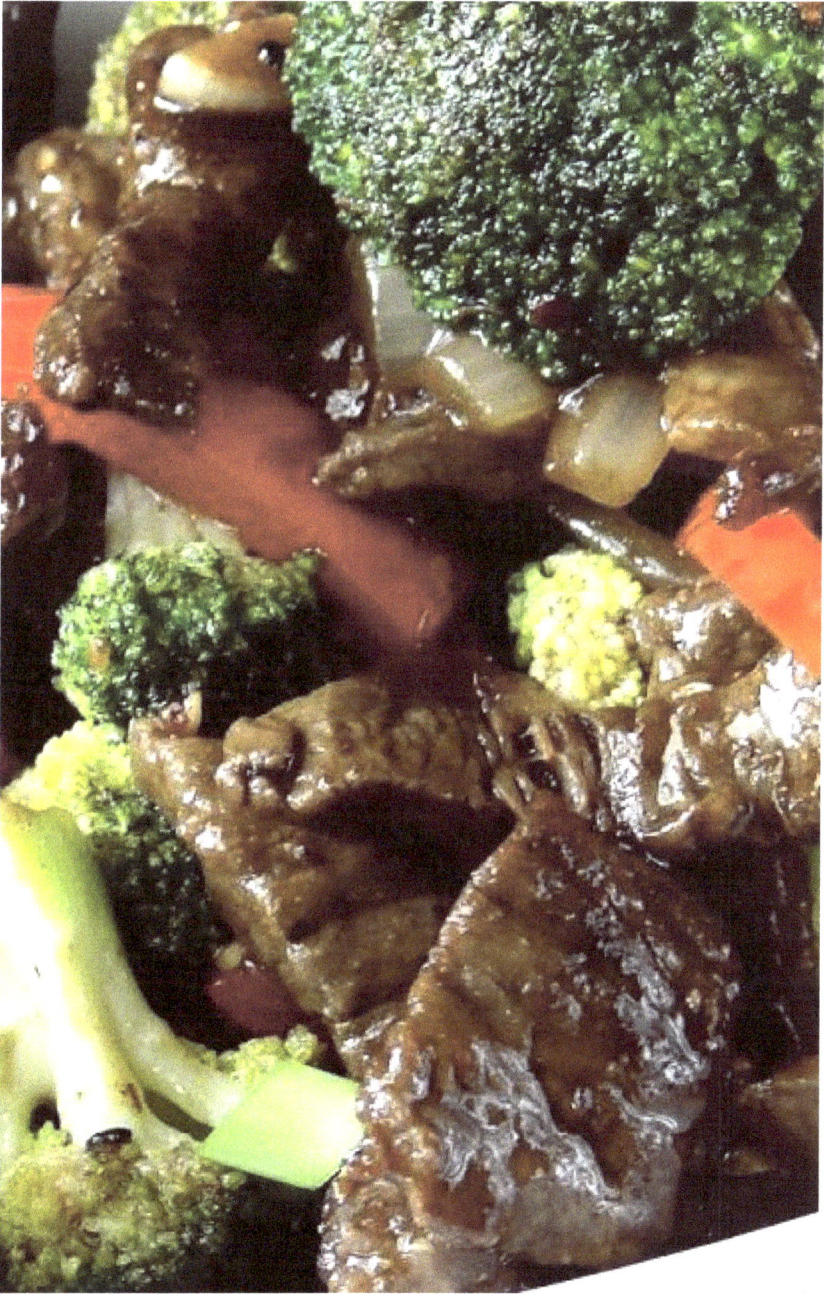

Pesto Chicken and Veggies

Preparation Time: 10 minutes

Cooking Time: 35 minutes

Serving: 3

Ingredients:

- 2 tbsp. olive oil
- 1 cup cherry tomatoes
- ¼ cup basil pesto
- 1/3 cup sun-dried tomatoes
- 1-pound chicken thigh
- 1-pound asparagus

Directions:

1. Preheat two tablespoons of olive oil and sliced chicken on medium heat. Season and add ½ cup of the sun-dried tomatoes.
2. Cook well. Spoon out the chicken and tomatoes and put them in a separate container.
3. Place the asparagus in same skillet and pour in the pesto. Put heat on medium and add the remaining sun-dried tomatoes. Cook for 10 minutes. Put it on a separate plate.
4. Position the chicken back in the pan and pour in pesto. Stir over medium heat for 2 minutes.

Nutrition:

- 104 calories
- 8g fat
- 26g protein

Crispy Peanut Tofu and Cauliflower Rice Stir-Fry

Preparation Time: 10 minutes

Cooking Time: 80 minutes

Serving: 4

Ingredients:

- 12 oz. tofu
- 1 tbsp. sesame oil
- 2 cloves garlic
- 1 small cauliflower head

For the sauce:

- 1 ½ tbsp. sesame oil
- ½ tsp. chili garlic sauce
- 2 ½ tbsp. peanut butter
- ¼ cup low sodium soy sauce
- ½ cup light brown sugar

Directions:

1. Strain tofu for 90 minutes.
2. Preheat the oven to 400 degrees Fahrenheit. Cube the tofu, and prepare your baking sheet.
3. Bake for 25 minutes and allow it to cool.
4. Combine the sauce ingredients.

5. Put the tofu in the sauce and coat the tofu thoroughly. Leave it for 15 minutes.

6. Shred the cauliflower into rice- size bits.

7. Situate skillet on medium heat. Cook veggies on a bit of sesame oil and soy sauce. Set aside.

8. Put tofu on the pan. Stir frequently. Set aside.

9. Steam your cauliflower rice for 8 minutes. Stir some sauce.

10. Mix ingredients together. Mix cauliflower rice with the veggies and tofu. Serve.

Nutrition:

- 107 calories
- 9g fat
- 30g protein

Keto Fried Chicken

Preparation Time: 10 minutes

Cooking Time: 45 minutes

Serving: 4

Ingredients:

- 4 chicken thighs
- Frying oil
- 2 large eggs
- 2 tbsp. heavy whipping cream

For the breading:

- 2/3 cup parmesan cheese
- 2/3 cup almond flour
- 1 tsp. salt
- ½ tsp. black pepper
- ½ tsp. cayenne
- ½ tsp. paprika

Directions:

1. Beat together the eggs and heavy cream.
2. Mix all the breading ingredients. Set aside.
3. Cut the chicken thigh into 3 even pieces and pat dry with paper towel.

4. Dip the chicken in the bread first before dipping it in the egg wash and then finally, dipping it in the breading again.
5. Fill 2 inches of oil in a pot and preheat at 350 degrees Fahrenheit. Gradually lower the heat.
6. Put the coated chicken in your hot oil. Fry for 5 minutes.
7. Strain cooked chicken.
8. Try not to overcrowd the pan. Serve.

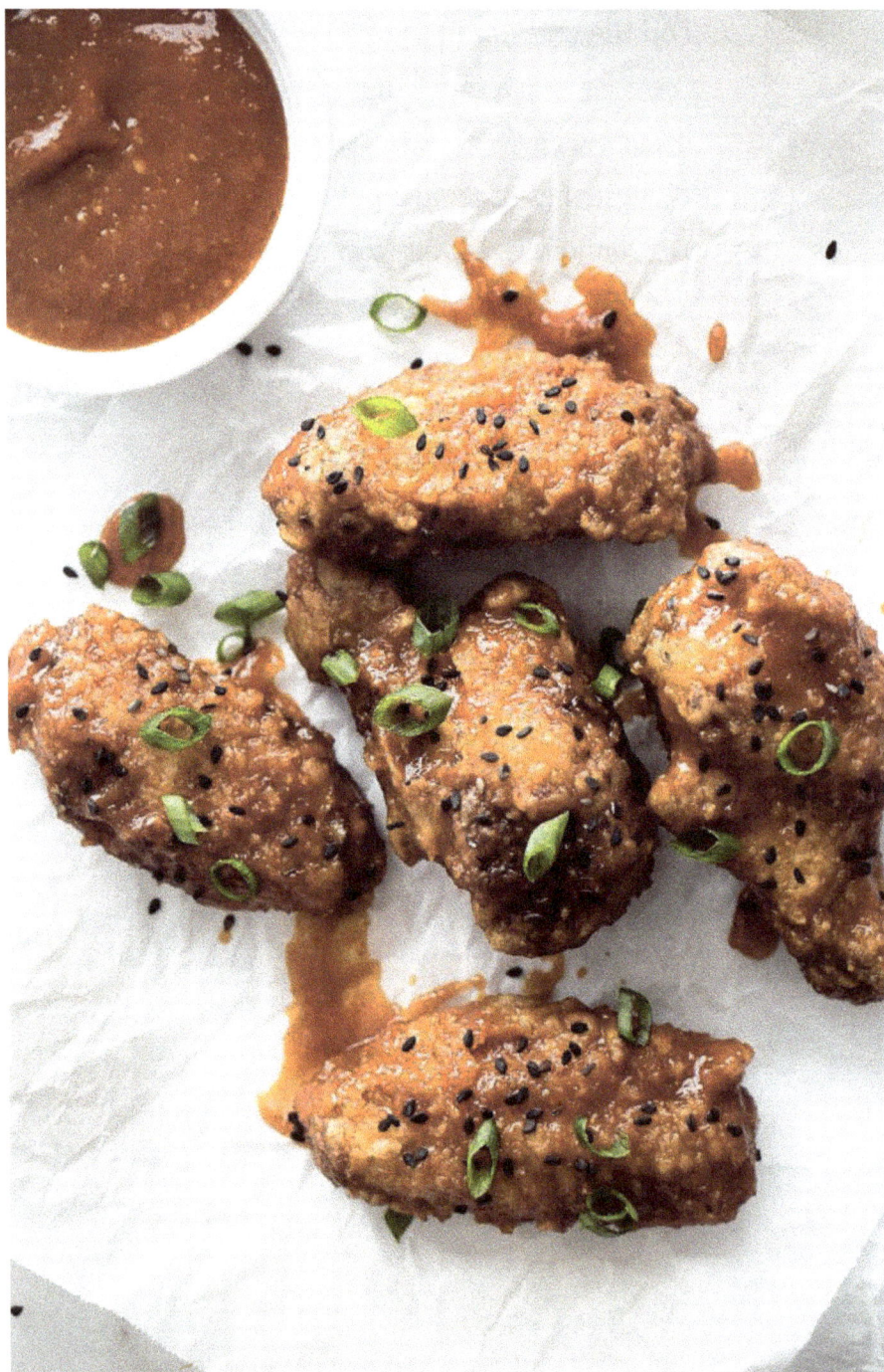

Roasted Cauliflower with Prosciutto, Capers, and Almonds

Preparation Time: 5 minutes

Cooking Time: 25 minutes

Servings: 2

Ingredients:

- 12 ounces cauliflower florets (I get precut florets at Trader Joe's)
- 2 tablespoons leftover bacon grease, or olive oil
- Pink Himalayan salt
- Freshly ground black pepper
- 2 ounces sliced prosciutto, torn into small pieces
- ¼ cup slivered almonds
- 2 tablespoons capers
- 2 tablespoons grated Parmesan cheese

Directions:

1. Preheat the oven to 400°F. Line a baking pan with a silicone baking mat or parchment paper. Put the cauliflower florets in the prepared baking pan with the bacon grease, and season with pink Himalayan salt and pepper. Or if you are using olive oil instead, drizzle

the cauliflower with olive oil and season with pink Himalayan salt and pepper.

2. Roast the cauliflower for 15 minutes. Stir the cauliflower so all sides are coated with the bacon grease. Distribute the prosciutto pieces in the pan.

3. Then add the slivered almonds and capers. Stir to combine. Sprinkle the Parmesan cheese on top, and roast for 10 minutes more.

4. Divide between two plates, using a slotted spoon so you don't get excess grease in the plates, and serve.

Nutrition:

- 288 Calories
- 24g Total Fat
- 7g Carbohydrates
- 14g Protein

Buttery Slow-Cooker Mushrooms

Preparation Time: 10 minutes

Cooking Time: 4 hours

Servings: 2

Ingredients:

- 6 tablespoons butter
- 1 tablespoon packaged dry ranch-dressing mix
- 8 ounces fresh cremini mushrooms
- 2 tablespoons grated Parmesan cheese
- 1 tablespoon chopped fresh flat-leaf Italian parsley

Directions:

1. With the crock insert in place, preheat the slow cooker to low. Put the butter and the dry ranch dressing in the bottom of the slow cooker, and allow the butter to melt. Stir to blend the dressing mix and butter.
2. Add the mushrooms to the slow cooker, and stir to coat with the butter-dressing mixture. Sprinkle the top with the Parmesan cheese. Cover and cook on low for 4 hours.
3. Use a slotted spoon to transfer the mushrooms to a serving dish. Top with the chopped parsley and serve.

Nutrition:

- 351 Calories
- 36g Total Fat
- 1g Fiber
- 6g Protein

Baked Zucchini Gratin

Preparation Time: 40 minutes

Cooking Time: 25 minutes

Servings: 2

Ingredients:

- 1 large zucchini, cut into ¼-inch-thick slices
- Pink Himalayan salt
- 1-ounce Brie cheese, rind trimmed off
- 1 tablespoon butter
- Freshly ground black pepper
- 1/3 cup shredded Gruyere cheese
- ¼ cup crushed pork rinds

Directions:

1. Salt the zucchini slices and put them in a colander in the sink for 45 minutes; the zucchini will shed much of their water. Preheat the oven to 400°F.
2. When the zucchini has been "weeping" for about 30 minutes, in a small saucepan over medium-low heat, heat the Brie and butter, stirring occasionally, until the cheese has melted and the mixture is fully combined, about 2 minutes.
3. Arrange the zucchini in an 8-inch baking dish so the zucchini slices are overlapping a bit. Season with

pepper. Pour the Brie mixture over the zucchini, and top with the shredded Gruyere cheese.

4. Sprinkle the crushed pork rinds over the top. Bake for about 25 minutes, until the dish is bubbling and the top is nicely browned, and serve.

Nutrition:

- 355 Calories
- 25g Total Fat
- 2g Fiber
- 28g Protein

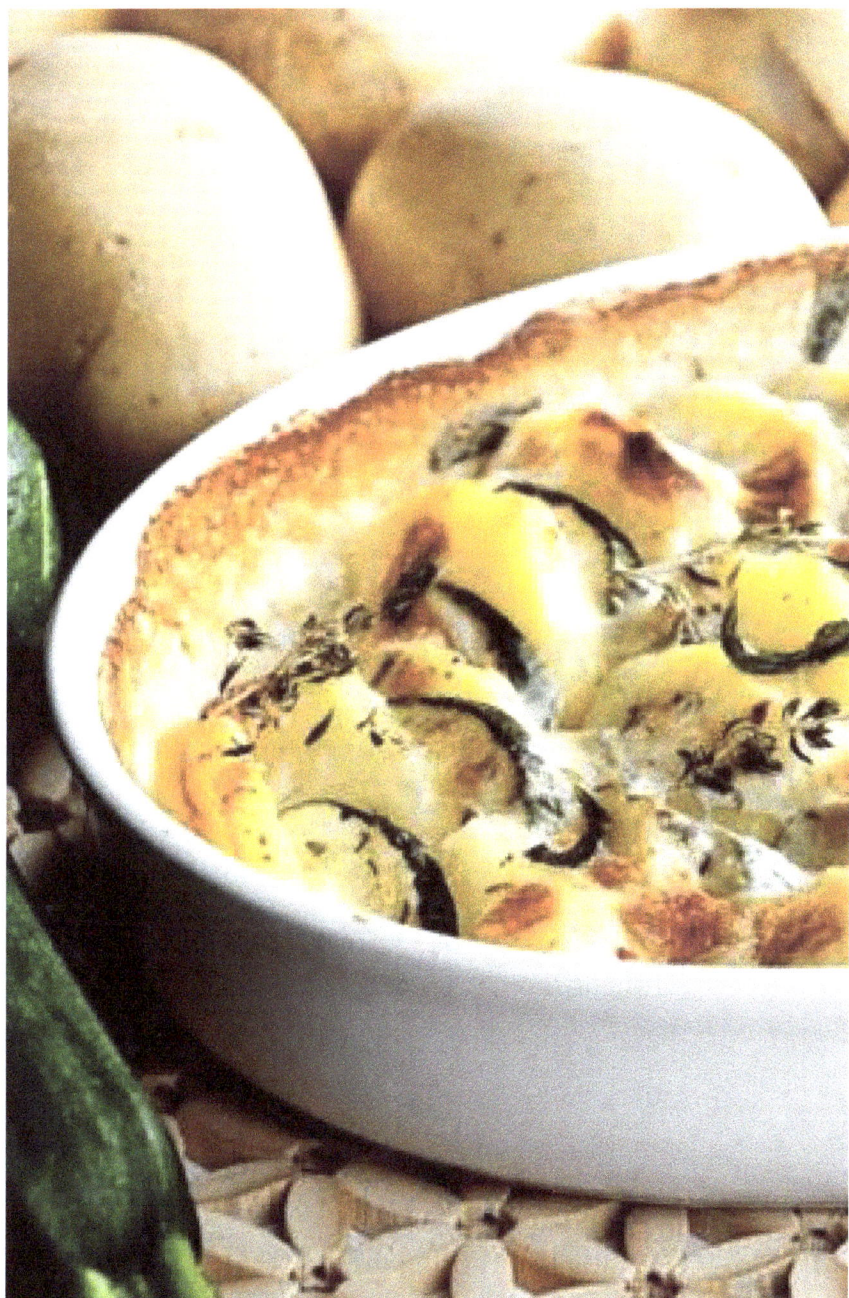

Roasted Radishes with Brown Butter Sauce

Preparation Time: 10 minutes

Cooking Time: 15 minutes

Servings: 2

Ingredients:

- 2 cups halved radishes
- 1 tablespoon olive oil
- Pink Himalayan salt
- Freshly ground black pepper
- 2 tablespoons butter
- 1 tablespoon chopped fresh flat-leaf Italian parsley

Directions:

1. Preheat the oven to 450°F. In a medium bowl, toss the radishes in the olive oil and season with pink Himalayan salt and pepper. Spread the radishes on a baking sheet in a single layer. Roast for 15 minutes, stirring halfway through.

2. Meanwhile, when the radishes have been roasting for about 10 minutes, in a small, light-colored saucepan over medium heat, melt the butter completely, stirring frequently, and season with pink Himalayan salt. When the butter begins to bubble and foam, continue

stirring. When the bubbling diminishes a bit, the butter should be a nice nutty brown. The browning process should take 3 minutes total. Transfer the browned butter to a heat-safe container (I use a mug).

3. Remove the radishes from the oven, and divide them between two plates. Spoon the brown butter over the radishes, top with the chopped parsley, and serve.

Nutrition:

- 181 Calories
- 19g Total Fat
- 2g Fiber
- 1g Protein

Parmesan and Pork Rind Green Beans

Preparation Time: 5 minutes

Cooking Time: 15 minutes

Servings: 2

Ingredients:

- ½ pound fresh green beans
- 2 tablespoons crushed pork rinds
- 2 tablespoons olive oil
- 1 tablespoon grated Parmesan cheese
- Pink Himalayan salt
- Freshly ground black pepper

Directions:

1. Preheat the oven to 400°F. In a medium bowl, combine the green beans, pork rinds, olive oil, and Parmesan cheese. Season with pink Himalayan salt and pepper, and toss until the beans are thoroughly coated.

2. Spread the bean mixture on a baking sheet in a single layer, and roast for about 15 minutes. At the halfway point, give the pan a little shake to move the beans around, or just give them a stir. Divide the beans between two plates and serve.

Nutrition:

- 175 Calories
- 15g Total Fat
- 3g Fiber
- 6g Protein

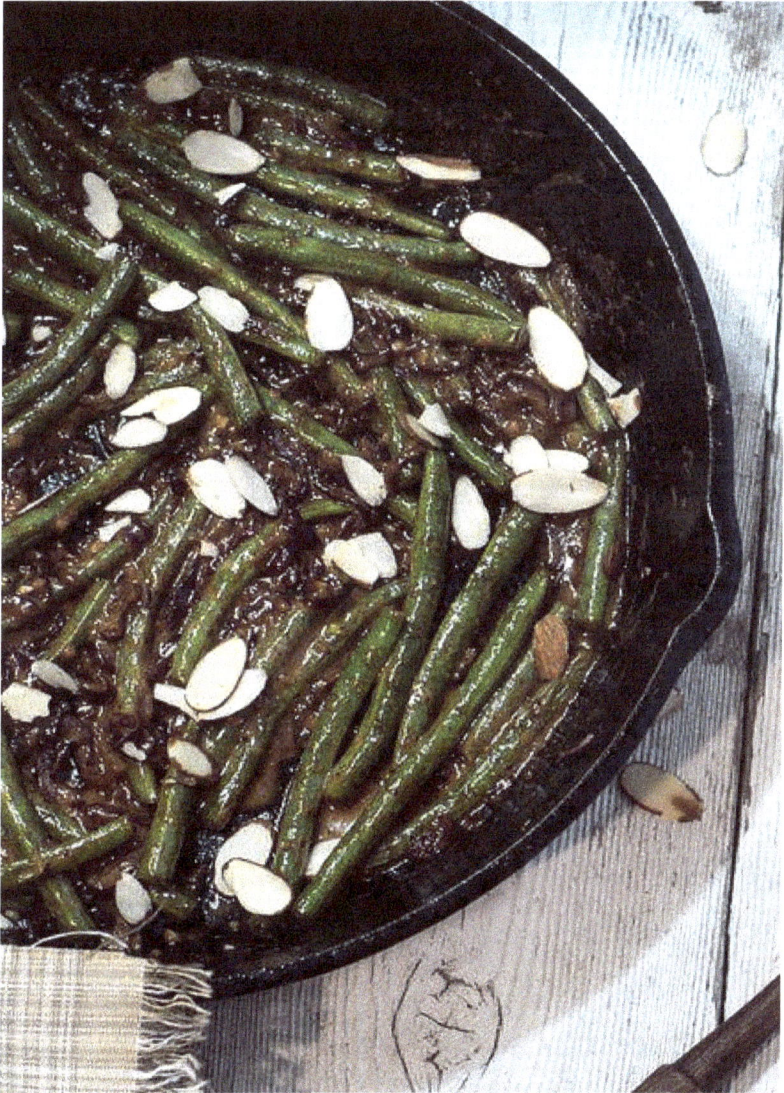

Pesto Cauliflower Steaks

Preparation Time: 5 minutes

Cooking Time: 20 minutes

Servings: 2

Ingredients:

- 2 tablespoons olive oil, plus more for brushing
- ½ head cauliflower
- Pink Himalayan salt
- Freshly ground black pepper
- 2 cups fresh basil leaves
- ½ cup grated Parmesan cheese
- ¼ cup almonds
- ½ cup shredded mozzarella cheese

Directions:

1. Preheat the oven to 425°F. Brush a baking sheet with olive oil or line with a silicone baking mat. To prep the cauliflower steaks, remove and discard the leaves and cut the cauliflower into 1-inch-thick slices. You can roast the extra floret crumbles that fall off with the steaks.

2. Place the cauliflower steaks on the prepared baking sheet, and brush them with the olive oil.

3. You want the surface just lightly coated so it gets caramelized. Season with pink Himalayan salt and pepper. Roast the cauliflower steaks for 20 minutes.

4. Meanwhile, put the basil, Parmesan cheese, almonds, and 2 tablespoons of olive oil in a food processor (or blender), and season with pink Himalayan salt and pepper. Mix until combined. Spread some pesto on top of each cauliflower steak, and top with the mozzarella cheese. Return to the oven and bake until the cheese melts, about 2 minutes. Place the cauliflower steaks on two plates, and serve hot.

Nutrition:

- 448 Calories
- 34g Total Fat
- 7g Fiber
- 24g Protein

Tomato, Avocado, and Cucumber Salad

Preparation Time: 5 minutes

Cooking Time: 5 minutes

Servings: 2

Ingredients:

- ½ cup grape tomatoes, halved
- 4 small Persian cucumbers or 1 English cucumber, peeled and finely chopped
- 1 avocado, finely chopped
- ¼ cup crumbled feta cheese
- 2 tablespoons vinaigrette salad dressing (I use Primal Kitchen Greek Vinaigrette)
- Pink Himalayan salt
- Freshly ground black pepper

Directions:

1. In a large bowl, combine the tomatoes, cucumbers, avocado, and feta cheese. Add the vinaigrette, and season with pink Himalayan salt and pepper. Toss to combine thoroughly. Divide the salad between two plates and serve.

Nutrition:

- 258 Calories
- 23g Total Fat
- 6g Fiber
- 5g Protein

Crunchy Pork Rind Zucchini Sticks

Preparation Time: 5 minutes

Cooking Time: 25 minutes

Servings: 2

Ingredients:

- 2 medium zucchinis, halved lengthwise and seeded
- ¼ cup crushed pork rinds
- ¼ cup grated Parmesan cheese
- 2 garlic cloves, minced
- 2 tablespoons melted butter
- Pink Himalayan salt
- Freshly ground black pepper
- Olive oil, for drizzling

Directions:

1. Preheat the oven to 400°F. Line a baking sheet with aluminum foil or a silicone baking mat. Place the zucchini halves cut-side up on the prepared baking sheet. In a medium bowl, combine the pork rinds, Parmesan cheese, garlic, and melted butter, and season with pink Himalayan salt and pepper. Mix until well combined.

2. Spoon the pork-rind mixture onto each zucchini stick, and drizzle each with a little olive oil. Bake for about

20 minutes, or until the topping is golden brown. Turn on the broiler to finish browning the zucchini sticks, 3 to 5 minutes, and serve.

Nutrition:

- 231 Calories
- 20g Total Fat
- 2g Fiber

Cheese Chips and Guacamole

Preparation Time: 10 minutes

Cooking Time: 10 minutes

Servings: 2

Ingredients:

For the Cheese Chips:

- 1 cup shredded cheese

For the Guacamole:

- 1 avocado, mashed
- Juice of ½ lime
- 1 teaspoon diced jalapeño
- 2 tablespoons chopped fresh cilantro leaves
- Pink Himalayan salt
- Freshly ground black pepper

Directions:

1. To Make the Cheese Chips
2. Preheat the oven to 350°F. Line a baking sheet with parchment paper or a silicone baking mat. Add ¼-cup mounds of shredded cheese to the pan, leaving plenty of space between them, and bake until the edges are brown and the middles have fully melted, about 7 minutes.

3. Set the pan on a cooling rack, and let the cheese chips cool for 5 minutes.
4. The chips will be floppy when they first come out of the oven but will crisp as they cool.
5. To Make the Guacamole
6. In a medium bowl, mix together the avocado, lime juice, jalapeño, and cilantro, and season with pink Himalayan salt and pepper. Top the cheese chips with the guacamole, and serve.

Nutrition:

- 323 Calories
- 27g Total Fat
- 5g Fiber
- 15g Protein

Cauliflower "Potato" Salad

Preparation Time: 10 minutes, plus 3 hours to chill

Cooking Time: 25 minutes

Servings: 2

Ingredients:

- ½ head cauliflower
- 1 tablespoon olive oil
- Pink Himalayan salt
- Freshly ground black pepper
- 1/3 cup mayonnaise
- 1 tablespoon mustard
- ¼ cup diced dill pickles
- 1 teaspoon paprika

Directions:

1. Preheat the oven to 400°F. Line a baking sheet with aluminum foil or a silicone baking mat. Cut the cauliflower into 1-inch pieces. Put the cauliflower in a large bowl, add the olive oil, season with the pink Himalayan salt and pepper, and toss to combine.

2. Spread the cauliflower out on the prepared baking sheet and bake for 25 minutes, or just until the cauliflower begins to brown. Halfway through the

cooking time, give the pan a couple of shakes or stir so all sides of the cauliflower cook.

3. In a large bowl, mix the cauliflower together with the mayonnaise, mustard, and pickles. Sprinkle the paprika on top, and chill in the refrigerator for 3 hours before serving.

Nutrition:

- 386 Calories
- 37g Total Fat
- 5g Fiber
- 5g Protein

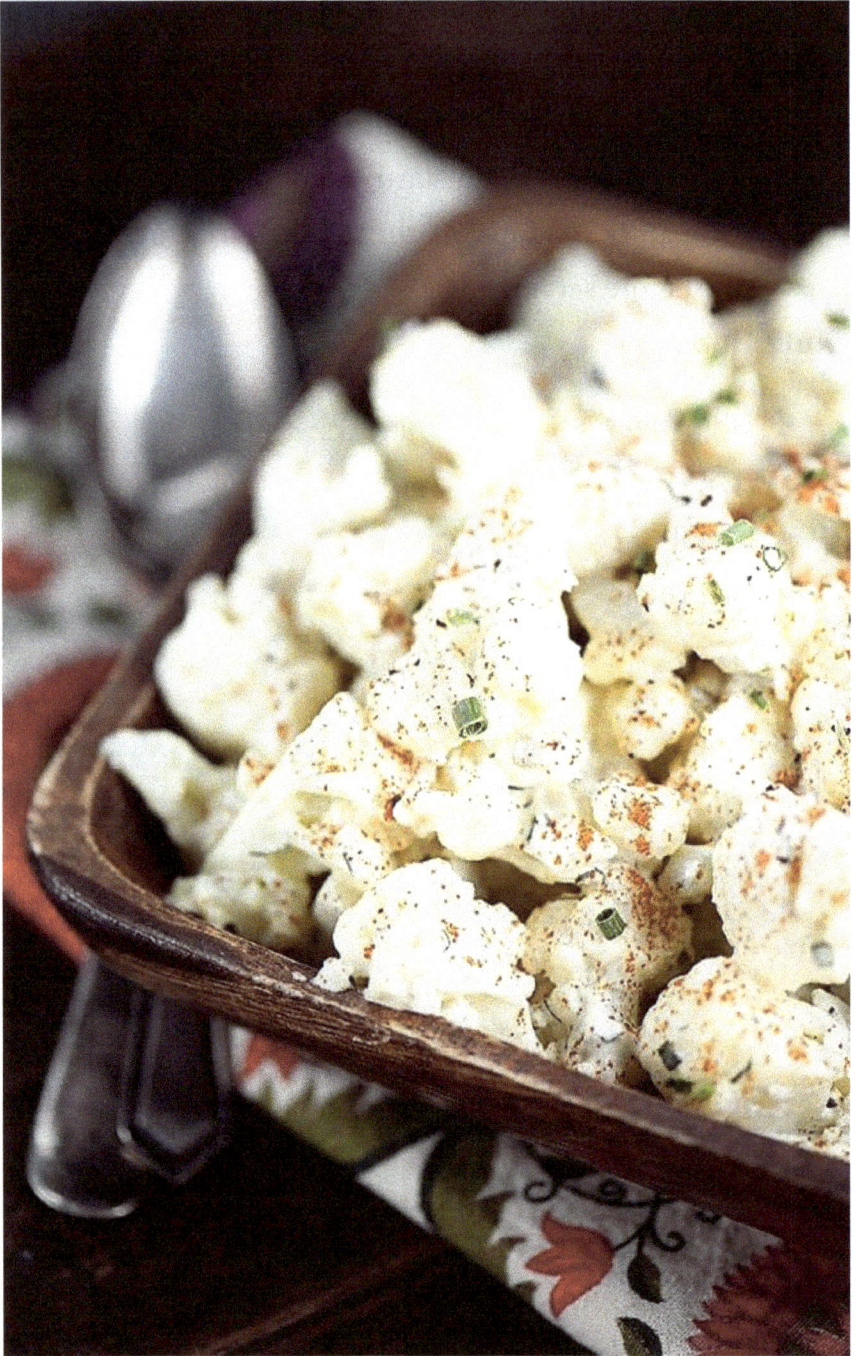

Loaded Cauliflower Mashed "Potatoes"

Preparation Time: 4 minutes

Cooking Time: 10 minutes

Servings: 4

Ingredients:

- 1 head fresh cauliflower, cut into cubes
- 2 garlic cloves, minced
- 6 tablespoons butter
- 2 tablespoons sour cream
- Pink Himalayan salt
- Freshly ground black pepper
- 1 cup shredded cheese (I use Colby Jack)
- 6 bacon slices, cooked and crumbled

Directions:

1. Boil a large pot of water over high heat. Add the cauliflower. Reduce the heat to medium-low and simmer for 8 to 10 minutes, until fork-tender. (You can also steam the cauliflower if you have a steamer basket.)

2. Drain the cauliflower in a colander, and turn it out onto a paper towel lined plate to soak up the water. Blot to remove any remaining water from the cauliflower pieces. This step is important; you want to

get out as much water as possible so the mash won't be runny.

3. Add the cauliflower to the food processor (or blender) with the garlic, butter, and sour cream, and season with pink Himalayan salt and pepper. Mix for about 1 minute, stopping to scrape down the sides of the bowl every 30 seconds.

4. Divide the cauliflower mix evenly among four small serving dishes, and top each with the cheese and bacon crumbles. (The cheese should melt from the hot cauliflower. But if you want to reheat it, you can put the cauliflower in oven-safe serving dishes and pop them under the broiler for 1 minute to heat up the cauliflower and melt the cheese.) Serve warm.

Nutrition:

- 757 Calories
- 38g Total Fat
- 6g Fiber
- 29g Protein

Low Carb Broccoli and Cheese Fritters

Preparation Time: 10 minutes

Cooking Time: 5 minutes

Servings: 16

Ingredients:

The Fritters:

- ¾ cup almond flour
- 7 tablespoons flaxseed meal
- 4 ounces fresh broccoli
- 4 ounces mozzarella cheese
- 2 large eggs
- 2 teaspoons baking powder
- Salt and Pepper to taste

The Sauce:

- ¼ cup mayonnaise
- ¼ cup fresh chopped dill
- ½ tablespoon lemon juice
- Salt and pepper to taste

Directions:

1. Add broccoli to a food processor and pulse until the broccoli is broken down into small pieces. You want it to be well processed. Mix together the cheese, almond

flour, ¼ cup flaxseed meal and baking powder with the broccoli.

2. If you want to add any extra seasonings (salt and pepper), do it at this point.

3. Add the 2 eggs and mix together well until everything is incorporated. Roll the batter into balls and then coat with 3 tablespoons flaxseed meal. Continue doing this with all of the batter and set aside on paper towels.

4. Heat your deep fat fryer to 375F. I use this deep fat fryer. Once ready, lay broccoli and cheese fritters inside the basket, not overcrowding it.

5. Fry the fritters until golden brown, about 3-5 minutes. Once done, lay on paper towels to drain excess grease and season to your tastes. Feel free to make a zesty dill and lemon mayonnaise for a dip. Enjoy!

Nutrition:

- 78 Calories
- 5.8g Fats
- 4.6g Protein

www.ingramcontent.com/pod-product-compliance
Lightning Source LLC
Chambersburg PA
CBHW050746030426
42336CB00012B/1680